Biohacking Your Genetic Potential

Unlocking the Secrets to a Healthier, Longer Life

Garth E. Wells

Table Of Contents

Table Of Contents

Introduction: The New Frontier of Health

Explore the future of biohacking, where cutting-edge science meets the timeless quest for optimal health and longevity. In this era, we are no longer passive recipients of generic health advice; instead, we become active participants in our well-being, leveraging personalized strategies tailored to our unique genetic makeup. This transformative approach is revolutionizing how we understand and pursue health, and it's opening doors to possibilities that were once the realm of science fiction.

The Evolution of Biohacking

Biohacking is a term that encompasses a wide range of practices aimed at enhancing physical and mental performance, improving health, and extending lifespan. While the concept might seem modern, its roots can be traced back to ancient times. Early practitioners of biohacking might not have had the technology we do today, but they were equally committed to understanding and optimizing their bodies. From ancient herbal remedies to the meditative practices of monks, the quest to push human limits has always been a part of our history.

Today, biohacking is fueled by advancements in genetics, biotechnology, and data science. The availability of genetic testing has been a game-changer, allowing individuals to gain insights into their DNA and understand how their genetic profile influences their health. This information empowers people to make informed decisions about their diet, exercise, and lifestyle, leading to more effective and personalized health strategies.

Personalization: The Key to Effective Biohacking

At the heart of the biohacking revolution is personalization. Traditional health advice often takes a one-size-fits-all approach, but the reality is that each person is unique. By understanding our genetic blueprint, we can tailor our health strategies to our specific needs, maximizing their effectiveness.

For example, genetic testing can reveal how your body responds to different types of food, your predisposition to certain health conditions, and your optimal exercise routines. Armed with this knowledge, you can create a personalized diet plan that supports your metabolism, a fitness regimen that aligns with your physical capabilities, and a lifestyle that promotes overall well-being.

The Integration of Technology

The integration of technology is another critical aspect of modern biohacking. Wearable devices, such as fitness trackers and smartwatches, provide real-time data on various health metrics, including heart rate, sleep patterns, and activity levels. This data can be used to monitor your progress, identify areas for improvement, and adjust your strategies accordingly.

Moreover, advancements in biotechnology are paving the way for more sophisticated biohacks. For instance, the development of nootropics – supplements designed to enhance cognitive function – offers the potential to boost mental performance and clarity. Similarly, innovations in personalized medicine, such as tailored drug therapies based on genetic profiles, are redefining how we approach treatment and prevention.

Challenges and Ethical Considerations

While the potential of biohacking is immense, it is not without challenges and ethical considerations. The accessibility of genetic information raises questions about privacy and data security. How can we ensure that our genetic data is protected and used responsibly? Furthermore, the rapid pace of technological advancement often outstrips regulatory frameworks, leading to concerns about safety and ethical standards.

It is crucial to approach biohacking with a balanced perspective, recognizing both its potential and its limitations. Ethical biohacking involves being informed, cautious, and responsible, always considering the long-term implications of our actions.

Embracing the Biohacking Lifestyle

As we embark on this journey into the new frontier of health, it is essential to cultivate a mindset of curiosity, experimentation, and continual learning. Biohacking is not a one-time event but a lifelong commitment to understanding and optimizing our bodies. By embracing this proactive approach, we can unlock the secrets to a healthier, longer life, pushing the boundaries of what is possible for human health and performance.

How Personalization is Changing the Game

In an era defined by technological advancement and scientific discovery, the concept of personalization is revolutionizing the health and wellness landscape. This paradigm shift from a one-size-fits-all approach to a more individualized strategy is transforming how we understand, manage, and optimize our health. Personalization is not just a trend; it's a game-changer that holds the potential to dramatically improve outcomes across various dimensions of health and wellness.

The Era of Personalized Medicine

At the forefront of this transformation is personalized medicine, which tailors medical treatment to the individual characteristics of each patient. This approach takes into account not only genetic information but also lifestyle, environment, and personal preferences. The advent of genomic sequencing has made it possible to identify genetic markers that can predict an individual's response to specific treatments. For example, pharmacogenomics studies how genes affect a person's response to drugs, allowing for the selection of medications that are most likely to be effective and cause the least side effects.

This shift towards personalized medicine is already having a profound impact on the treatment of diseases such as cancer. Oncologists can now use genetic testing to identify mutations in a patient's tumor and select targeted therapies that are more likely to be effective. This precision in treatment not only improves outcomes but also reduces the trial-and-error process that often accompanies traditional treatment methods.

Personalized Nutrition and Diet Plans

Personalization extends beyond medicine to everyday aspects of health, such as nutrition and diet. Traditional dietary guidelines provide general recommendations that may not be suitable for everyone. Personalized nutrition, on the other hand, uses genetic information, metabolic markers, and other personal data to create diet plans tailored to an individual's unique needs.

For instance, some people may have genetic variations that affect how they metabolize certain nutrients. Personalized nutrition can identify these variations and suggest dietary adjustments that optimize nutrient absorption and metabolic health. This approach can help manage and prevent conditions such as obesity, diabetes, and cardiovascular disease more effectively than generic diet plans.

Tailored Fitness Regimens

Fitness is another area where personalization is making significant strides. Personalized fitness regimens take into account an individual's genetic predispositions, physical capabilities, and personal goals. For example, genetic tests can reveal whether a person is more suited to endurance or strength training, allowing for a fitness plan that maximizes their potential.

Moreover, wearable technology and fitness apps provide real-time data on various metrics, such as heart rate, activity levels, and sleep patterns. This data can be used to monitor progress, make adjustments, and keep motivation high. Personalized fitness programs can also help prevent injuries by considering an individual's biomechanics and susceptibilities.

Mental Health and Cognitive Performance

The personalization trend is also transforming mental health care and cognitive performance optimization. Genetic tests and neuroimaging can provide insights into an individual's susceptibility to mental health disorders, response to different therapies, and cognitive strengths and weaknesses. This information allows for the creation of personalized mental health care plans that are more effective and sustainable.

For instance, personalized approaches can identify the most suitable types of therapy (such as cognitive-behavioral therapy or mindfulness-based therapy) and even suggest specific lifestyle changes to improve mental health. Similarly, nootropics – substances that enhance cognitive function – can be tailored to individual needs, optimizing brain performance and mental clarity.

Wearable Technology and Health Tracking

Wearable technology is a powerful tool in the personalization arsenal. Devices like fitness trackers, smartwatches, and health monitoring apps collect vast amounts of data on an individual's daily activities, physiological responses, and sleep patterns. This data provides valuable insights that can be used to fine-tune health strategies.

For example, by analyzing sleep patterns, individuals can identify factors that impact their sleep quality and make necessary adjustments. Similarly, tracking daily activity levels and physiological responses helps optimize workout routines and monitor overall health.

The continuous feedback loop provided by wearable technology ensures that health strategies are always aligned with an individual's current state and goals.

The Future of Personalization in Health

The potential of personalization in health and wellness is vast and continually expanding. As technology advances and our understanding of the human body deepens, the opportunities for individualized health strategies will only grow. Future developments may include more sophisticated genetic testing, advanced wearable technologies, and AI-driven health analytics, further enhancing the precision and effectiveness of personalized health care.

Chapter 1: Decoding Your DNA

The concept of decoding your DNA may sound like something out of a science fiction novel, but it's very much a reality today. Advancements in genetic testing and biotechnology have made it possible for individuals to unlock the secrets hidden within their genetic code. This chapter explores the science behind genetic testing, the process of understanding your genetic blueprint, and the practical applications of this knowledge in optimizing health and wellness.

The Science Behind Genetic Testing

Genetic testing involves analyzing your DNA, the molecule that carries the genetic instructions used in the growth, development, and functioning of all living organisms. DNA is composed of sequences of four nucleotides—adenine (A), thymine (T), cytosine (C), and guanine (G)—arranged in a double helix structure. The human genome contains about 3 billion of these nucleotide pairs, which make up thousands of genes.

Each gene contains specific instructions for producing proteins, which perform most of the biological functions in our bodies. Variations in these genes, known as polymorphisms or mutations, can influence everything from your eye color to your risk for certain diseases. Genetic testing identifies these variations, providing valuable insights into your unique genetic makeup.

There are several types of genetic tests, including whole genome sequencing, which reads the entire DNA sequence, and more targeted tests, which focus on specific genes or regions associated with particular traits or health conditions. Advances in technology have made these tests more accessible and affordable, allowing individuals to gain detailed knowledge about their genetic predispositions.

Understanding Your Genetic Blueprint

Decoding your DNA starts with understanding your genetic blueprint. This blueprint is like an instruction manual for your body, outlining how your cells should function and respond to various stimuli. By analyzing your genetic information, you can gain insights into several aspects of your health and wellness:

1. Health Risks and Predispositions: Genetic testing can reveal your predisposition to various health conditions, such as heart disease, diabetes, cancer, and autoimmune disorders. This information can help you take proactive measures to monitor and mitigate these risks.

2. Nutritional Needs: Your genes influence how your body processes and utilizes nutrients. Genetic testing can identify specific dietary needs and intolerances, allowing you to tailor your nutrition for optimal health.

3. Fitness and Exercise: Your genetic profile can indicate how your body responds to different types of exercise, such as endurance training or strength training. This knowledge can help you design a fitness regimen that maximizes your performance and reduces the risk of injury.

4. Drug Response: Pharmacogenomics, the study of how genes affect your response to drugs, can guide personalized medication choices. By understanding your genetic makeup, healthcare providers can select medications that are most likely to be effective and have the fewest side effects.

5. Behavioral Traits: Genes also play a role in shaping your behavior, including your tendencies towards stress, addiction, and mental health conditions. Genetic insights can inform strategies for managing mental health and improving emotional well-being.

Practical Applications of Genetic Knowledge

Once you have decoded your DNA, the real power lies in applying this knowledge to enhance your health and wellness. Here are some practical ways to leverage your genetic information:

1. Personalized Health Plans: Create a comprehensive health plan tailored to your genetic profile. This plan can include specific dietary recommendations, exercise routines, and lifestyle modifications designed to optimize your health.

2. Preventive Measures: Use genetic insights to adopt preventive measures against potential health risks. For example, if you have a genetic predisposition to heart disease, you can focus on heart-healthy habits, such as maintaining a balanced diet, exercising regularly, and managing stress.

3. Customized Nutrition: Develop a personalized nutrition plan based on your genetic needs. This plan can help you avoid foods that your body doesn't tolerate well and incorporate nutrients that your body requires for optimal function.

4. Optimized Fitness: Design a fitness program that aligns with your genetic strengths and weaknesses. Whether you're more suited to endurance sports or strength training, personalized fitness can enhance your performance and reduce the risk of injury.

5. Targeted Therapies: In the realm of medicine, genetic testing can guide the selection of targeted therapies. For conditions like cancer, personalized treatment plans based on genetic mutations can significantly improve outcomes.

Ethical Considerations and Privacy

Genetic testing provides many advantages, but it also poses significant ethical and privacy issues that need to be carefully considered. Genetic information is highly sensitive, and there are risks associated with its misuse.

It is essential to ensure that genetic data is stored securely and used responsibly. Considerations around genetic discrimination in employment and insurance also need to be addressed.

Case Study: Real-Life Genetic Success

Personalized medicine, fueled by advancements in genetic testing, is transforming healthcare. Real-life stories of individuals who have benefited from these advancements illustrate the profound impact of understanding and utilizing genetic information. This case study explores several such success stories, highlighting how genetic insights have led to improved health outcomes, personalized treatments, and enhanced quality of life.

Case Study 1: Predicting and Preventing Breast Cancer

Sarah, a 42-year-old mother of two, decided to undergo genetic testing after her mother and grandmother both battled breast cancer. Her genetic test revealed a

BRCA1 mutation, significantly increasing her risk of developing breast and ovarian cancer. Armed with this information, Sarah took proactive measures to manage her risk.

With guidance from her healthcare team, Sarah opted for enhanced surveillance, including regular mammograms and MRIs, to catch any signs of cancer early. She also chose to undergo prophylactic surgeries, including a double mastectomy and an oophorectomy, which drastically reduced her risk of developing cancer. By understanding her genetic predisposition, Sarah not only took control of her health but also provided invaluable information for her daughters, who can now make informed decisions about their own health in the future.

Case Study 2: Tailoring Treatment for Cystic Fibrosis

Tom, a young boy diagnosed with cystic fibrosis (CF), faced numerous challenges due to the chronic and progressive nature of the disease. Traditional treatments focused on managing symptoms rather than addressing the underlying genetic cause. However, genetic testing identified the specific mutations in Tom's CFTR gene responsible for his condition.

This information allowed his medical team to prescribe a new class of medications called CFTR modulators, designed to target the defective protein produced by the CFTR gene mutations. The personalized treatment plan significantly improved Tom's lung function, reduced hospitalizations, and enhanced his overall quality of life. Genetic insights enabled a shift from symptom management to targeted therapy, offering Tom a brighter and healthier future.

Case Study 3: Optimizing Mental Health

Emily, a 28-year-old professional, struggled with anxiety and depression for years. Despite trying various medications, she found limited relief and often experienced adverse side effects. Frustrated and desperate for a solution, Emily underwent pharmacogenomic testing to understand how her genetic makeup influenced her response to psychiatric medications.

The test results revealed that Emily had specific genetic variations affecting the metabolism of certain antidepressants. Armed with this knowledge, her psychiatrist was able to prescribe medications that were more likely to be effective and cause fewer side effects. Within weeks, Emily noticed a significant improvement in her mood and anxiety levels. This personalized approach to mental health treatment not only alleviated her symptoms but also restored her hope and confidence in managing her condition.

Case Study 4: Managing Diabetes with Personalized Nutrition

John, a 50-year-old man with a family history of diabetes, was diagnosed with type 2 diabetes. Despite following general dietary guidelines and medication regimens, he struggled to control his blood sugar levels. Determined to find a better solution, John underwent genetic testing to explore how his body responded to different nutrients and foods.

The test revealed that John had genetic variations affecting his carbohydrate metabolism and insulin sensitivity. With the help of a genetic nutritionist, John developed a personalized meal plan tailored to his genetic profile. By adjusting his diet to include more protein, healthy fats, and specific carbohydrates, he was able to stabilize his blood sugar levels, reduce his medication dosage, and achieve a healthier weight. The personalized nutrition plan transformed John's approach to managing diabetes, significantly improving his health and quality of life.

Case Study 5: Enhancing Athletic Performance

Mark, a 25-year-old aspiring athlete, sought to optimize his training and performance. Despite rigorous training schedules, he felt he was not reaching his full potential. Genetic testing provided insights into his muscle composition, endurance capacity, and injury risk.

The results indicated that Mark had a genetic predisposition for strength and power-based activities rather than endurance sports. With this information, Mark and his coach redesigned his training regimen to focus on weightlifting, sprinting, and high-intensity interval training (HIIT). Additionally, genetic insights into his recovery needs helped him incorporate personalized strategies for rest and nutrition.

Over time, Mark's performance improved significantly. He achieved personal bests in sprinting events and powerlifting competitions. The personalized training plan, informed by genetic testing, allowed Mark to unlock his full athletic potential and achieve his goals.

Case Study 6: Addressing Rare Genetic Disorders

Jane, a 10-year-old girl, exhibited developmental delays and a range of unexplained symptoms. After years of inconclusive tests and misdiagnoses, her parents pursued whole exome sequencing (WES) to identify the underlying cause. The genetic test revealed a rare mutation associated with a condition called Rett syndrome, a neurodevelopmental disorder that primarily affects girls.

With a definitive diagnosis, Jane's healthcare team could tailor her treatment and support strategies to her specific needs. Genetic counseling provided her family with a better understanding of the condition and guidance on managing her symptoms. Access to specialized therapies and interventions improved Jane's quality of life, enabling her to reach developmental milestones and participate more actively in daily activities. The genetic diagnosis provided clarity and direction, transforming Jane's care and offering hope for the future.

Chapter 2: Personalized Nutrition for Optimal Health

Nutrition is a crucial cornerstone in the pursuit of overall wellness. The foods we consume not only fuel our bodies but also influence our overall well-being, disease susceptibility, and longevity. While general dietary guidelines offer a broad approach to healthy eating, personalized nutrition tailors dietary recommendations to an individual's unique genetic makeup, lifestyle, and health needs. This chapter delves into the concept of personalized nutrition, its scientific foundations, and its transformative potential for achieving optimal health.

The Science of Personalized Nutrition

Personalized nutrition, also known as precision nutrition, is based on the understanding that each individual has a unique set of genetic, environmental, and lifestyle factors that influence their nutritional needs and responses to different foods. By analyzing an individual's genetic information, along with other biomarkers, personalized nutrition aims to provide dietary recommendations that are specifically designed to optimize health outcomes.

Genetic Influences on Nutrition

Our genes play a crucial role in determining how our bodies metabolize and respond to nutrients. For instance, variations in certain genes can affect how efficiently we process macronutrients (carbohydrates, fats, and proteins), absorb vitamins and minerals, and respond to bioactive compounds in foods. Here are some key areas where genetics impact nutrition:

1. **Macronutrient Metabolism:** Some individuals have genetic variations that make them more efficient at metabolizing carbohydrates, while others may process fats or proteins more effectively. Understanding these genetic differences can help tailor macronutrient intake to suit individual needs, potentially enhancing energy levels, weight management, and overall metabolic health.

2. Micronutrient Absorption: Genetic variations can also influence how well we absorb and utilize vitamins and minerals. For example, some people may have a higher requirement for vitamin D due to genetic factors affecting its metabolism, while others might need more folate or vitamin B12. Personalized nutrition can identify these needs and ensure adequate intake through diet or supplementation.

3. Food Sensitivities and Intolerances: Certain genetic markers are associated with sensitivities or intolerances to specific foods, such as lactose intolerance or gluten sensitivity. By identifying these genetic predispositions, personalized nutrition can help individuals avoid foods that may cause adverse reactions and discomfort.

4. Taste Preferences and Eating Behaviors: Genetics can also influence taste preferences and eating behaviors. For example, variations in taste receptor genes can affect sensitivity to bitter or sweet tastes, potentially impacting food choices and dietary habits. Personalized nutrition can account for these preferences, making healthy eating more enjoyable and sustainable.

Personalized Nutrition in Practice

Implementing personalized nutrition involves several steps, starting with the collection of genetic and lifestyle information, followed by the development of tailored dietary recommendations. Here's how the process typically works:

1. **Genetic Testing:** The first step in personalized nutrition is genetic testing, which involves analyzing DNA to identify genetic variations related to nutrition and metabolism. This can be done through a simple saliva or blood sample, which is then processed by a laboratory.

2. **Assessment of Lifestyle and Health Factors:** In addition to genetic information, personalized nutrition takes into account an individual's lifestyle, health status, and dietary habits. This comprehensive assessment helps create a more accurate and holistic nutritional plan.

3. **Development of a Personalized Nutrition Plan:** Based on the genetic and lifestyle data, a personalized nutrition plan is developed. This plan includes specific dietary recommendations, such as optimal macronutrient ratios, suggested foods and nutrients, and

guidance on managing any food sensitivities or intolerances.

4. Monitoring and Adjustments: Personalized nutrition is an ongoing process that involves regular monitoring and adjustments. As individuals' health status and lifestyle change, their nutritional needs may also evolve. Continuous feedback and updates ensure that the personalized nutrition plan remains effective and relevant.

Benefits of Personalized Nutrition

Personalized nutrition offers numerous benefits over traditional, one-size-fits-all dietary guidelines. Some of the main benefits include:

1. Improved Health Outcomes: By tailoring dietary recommendations to an individual's genetic profile, personalized nutrition can help prevent and manage chronic diseases, such as diabetes, cardiovascular disease, and obesity. Optimized nutrient intake supports overall health and well-being.

2. Enhanced Weight Management: Personalized nutrition can identify the most effective dietary strategies for weight management based on an individual's genetic predispositions. This targeted approach can lead to more sustainable and successful weight loss or maintenance.

3. Greater Nutrient Absorption: Understanding genetic variations in nutrient metabolism allows for more precise recommendations regarding vitamin and mineral intake. This ensures that individuals receive adequate nutrients to support their body's functions and prevent deficiencies.

4. Reduced Risk of Food Sensitivities: By identifying genetic predispositions to food sensitivities or intolerances, personalized nutrition can help individuals avoid foods that may cause adverse reactions, leading to improved digestive health and overall comfort.

5. Increased Motivation and Adherence: Personalized nutrition plans are tailored to individual preferences and needs, making them more enjoyable and easier to follow. This personalized approach can increase motivation and adherence to healthy eating habits.

Case Study: Personalized Nutrition Success

To illustrate the impact of personalized nutrition, consider the case of Laura, a 35-year-old woman struggling with weight management and fatigue. Despite following various diets, she found it challenging to achieve her health goals. After undergoing genetic testing, Laura discovered that she had a genetic variation affecting carbohydrate metabolism, making her more prone to weight gain when consuming a high-carbohydrate diet.

With the help of a nutritionist, Laura developed a personalized nutrition plan that reduced her carbohydrate intake and increased her consumption of healthy fats and proteins. She also identified a vitamin D deficiency due to genetic factors and began taking a supplement. Within a few months, Laura experienced significant improvements in her energy levels, mood, and weight management. The personalized nutrition plan helped her achieve her health goals in a way that generic diets had not.

Challenges and Future Directions

While personalized nutrition holds great promise, there are also challenges to consider. One major challenge is the accessibility and affordability of genetic testing and personalized nutrition services. As technology advances and becomes more widespread, it is hoped that these services will become more accessible to a broader population.

Tailoring Your Diet to Your DNA

The field of nutrition has undergone a remarkable transformation with the advent of genetic testing and personalized health. One of the most exciting developments in this area is the ability to tailor diets to an individual's DNA. This approach moves beyond generic dietary recommendations, offering personalized nutrition plans that take into account unique genetic variations. By understanding how our genetic makeup influences our nutritional needs and responses to different foods, we can optimize our diet for better health and wellness.

Understanding the Basics of Genetic Influence on Nutrition

Our genes play a significant role in determining how we metabolize nutrients, our risk of developing certain diseases, and our overall health. Genetic variations, known as single nucleotide polymorphisms (SNPs), can affect everything from nutrient absorption to metabolic efficiency. For example, some people may have genetic variants that make them more efficient at metabolizing fats, while others may process carbohydrates better. Knowing your genetic predispositions can inform personalized dietary advice that suits your individual requirements.

The Process of Tailoring Your Diet to Your DNA

1. Genetic Testing: The first step in tailoring your diet to your DNA is undergoing genetic testing. This usually involves providing a saliva or blood sample, which is then analyzed to identify specific genetic variants related to nutrition and metabolism. Several companies offer direct-to-consumer genetic testing kits, making it easier for individuals to access this information.

2. Interpreting the Results: Once the genetic data is available, the next step is interpreting the results. This often involves working with a healthcare provider or a genetic nutritionist who can explain what the genetic variations mean for your diet and health. They can help identify which nutrients your body needs more of, which foods to avoid, and how to adjust your macronutrient ratios.

3. Developing a Personalized Nutrition Plan: Based on the genetic insights, a personalized nutrition plan is created. This plan takes into account not only genetic predispositions but also lifestyle factors, health goals, and personal preferences. The goal is to create a sustainable and enjoyable diet that supports optimal health.

Key Areas Where DNA Influences Diet

1. Macronutrient Metabolism: One of the primary ways DNA influences diet is through macronutrient metabolism. For instance, some individuals may have a genetic predisposition to process carbohydrates more efficiently, making them better suited for a diet higher in carbohydrates. Others may have genes that favor fat metabolism, indicating that a higher-fat, lower-carb diet could be more effective for them.

2. Micronutrient Needs: Genetic variations can also affect how well we absorb and utilize vitamins and minerals. For example, some people may have a genetic variant that reduces their ability to absorb vitamin D, necessitating higher intake from food or supplements. Similarly, genetic testing can reveal predispositions to deficiencies in nutrients like iron, folate, or vitamin B12, allowing for targeted dietary adjustments.

3. Food Sensitivities and Intolerances: Genetic testing can identify predispositions to food sensitivities or intolerances. Common examples include lactose intolerance, gluten sensitivity, and histamine intolerance. Knowing about these genetic tendencies can help individuals avoid foods that may cause adverse reactions, improving digestive health and overall well-being.

4. Weight Management: Genetics can influence how the body stores and burns fat, affecting weight management. Some people may have genetic variants that make them more prone to weight gain, even with a healthy diet and regular exercise. Understanding these genetic factors can help tailor weight management strategies, such as adjusting macronutrient intake or incorporating specific types of physical activity.

Real-World Applications and Benefits

The real-world applications of tailoring your diet to your DNA are vast and varied. Here are some of the key benefits:

1. Improved Health Outcomes: By aligning dietary choices with genetic predispositions, individuals can improve their overall health. This approach can help prevent chronic diseases, manage existing conditions, and promote long-term wellness.

2. Enhanced Energy and Performance: Personalized nutrition can optimize nutrient intake, leading to better energy levels, enhanced athletic performance, and improved cognitive function. This is particularly beneficial for athletes and individuals with demanding lifestyles.

3. Better Weight Management: Tailoring diet to DNA can lead to more effective and sustainable weight management. By understanding how your body responds to different foods, you can create a diet that supports healthy weight loss or maintenance.

4. Increased Adherence to Healthy Eating: Personalized nutrition plans are designed to fit individual preferences and needs, making them easier to follow. This increases the likelihood of long-term adherence to healthy eating habits.

Challenges and Considerations

While the benefits of tailoring your diet to your DNA are substantial, there are also challenges and considerations. Genetic testing and personalized nutrition services can be costly and may not be accessible to everyone. Additionally, genetic information is complex and requires careful interpretation by trained professionals. There is also the need for ongoing research to fully understand the implications of various genetic variations on nutrition and health.

Meal Plans and Recipes for Genetic Optimization

Creating meal plans and recipes that align with your genetic makeup is a powerful way to enhance health and wellness. Genetic optimization through personalized nutrition helps individuals make informed dietary choices based on their unique genetic profile, leading to better health outcomes, increased energy, and overall well-being. This chapter explores the principles of designing meal plans and recipes tailored to genetic information, providing practical examples and tips for integrating this approach into everyday life.

Understanding Genetic Influences on Diet

Genetic testing can reveal a wealth of information about how our bodies process different nutrients, which foods may be beneficial or detrimental, and what dietary patterns best support our health. Key areas influenced by genetics include macronutrient metabolism (how we process proteins, fats, and carbohydrates), micronutrient needs (vitamins and minerals), food sensitivities and intolerances, and metabolic tendencies (such as propensity for weight gain or cholesterol levels). By tailoring meal plans to these genetic insights, individuals can optimize their nutrition to support their unique health needs.

Designing a Personalized Meal Plan

1. Assess Genetic Data: Begin by analyzing your genetic test results to understand your specific dietary needs. Look for insights on macronutrient metabolism, micronutrient requirements, and any identified food sensitivities or intolerances.

2. Set Nutritional Goals: Based on the genetic data, set clear nutritional goals. These might include optimizing energy levels, managing weight, supporting heart health, or improving digestive health. Personalized goals will guide the creation of your meal plan.

3. Plan Balanced Meals: Ensure each meal includes a balance of macronutrients tailored to your genetic profile. For example, if your genetics indicate a higher efficiency in metabolizing fats, include healthy fats like avocados, nuts, and olive oil. If you process carbohydrates well, focus on complex carbs like whole grains, fruits, and vegetables.

4. Incorporate Key Micronutrients: Identify any specific micronutrient needs highlighted by your genetic test. For example, if you have a higher requirement for vitamin D or B12, incorporate foods rich in these nutrients or consider supplementation as advised by a healthcare professional.

5. Address Food Sensitivities: Avoid foods that may trigger sensitivities or intolerances based on your genetic predispositions. Substitute with alternatives that provide similar nutritional benefits without causing adverse reactions.

Sample Meal Plan for Genetic Optimization

Breakfast: Energizing Smoothie Bowl

Ingredients:

- 1 cup spinach (rich in iron and folate)
- 1 banana (source of potassium)
- Mix together 1/2 cup of protein-rich Greek yogurt, which also contains beneficial probiotics,

and 1 tablespoon of chia seeds, a rich source of omega-3 fatty acids.

- 1/2 cup mixed berries (high in antioxidants)
- 1/2 cup almond milk (dairy alternative for those with lactose intolerance)

Instructions:

- Blend all ingredients until smooth.
- Pour into a bowl and top with sliced almonds and fresh berries.

Lunch: Quinoa Salad with Grilled Chicken

Ingredients:

- 1 cup cooked quinoa (complex carbohydrate and protein source)
- 1 serving of grilled chicken breast, an excellent source of protein
- 1/2 cup cherry tomatoes (rich in vitamins A and C)
- 1/2 cucumber, diced (hydrating and low in calories)
- 1/4 cup feta cheese (optional, for calcium)
- 1 tablespoon olive oil (healthy fat)
- Juice of 1 lemon (vitamin C boost)

- Salt and pepper to taste

Instructions:

- Combine quinoa, grilled chicken, cherry tomatoes, and cucumber in a bowl.
- Drizzle with olive oil and lemon juice.
- Season with salt and pepper and toss gently.

Snack: Apple Slices with Almond Butter

Ingredients:

- 1 apple, sliced (fiber and antioxidants)
- 2 tablespoons almond butter (healthy fat and protein)

Instructions:

- Dip apple slices in almond butter for a satisfying, nutrient-rich snack.

Dinner: Baked Salmon with Sweet Potato and Asparagus

Ingredients:

- 1 salmon filet (rich in omega-3 fatty acids)
- 1 sweet potato, cubed (complex carbohydrate and vitamin A)

- 1 bunch asparagus (fiber and folate)
- 1 tablespoon olive oil (healthy fat)
- Salt, pepper, and herbs to taste (flavor and additional nutrients)

Instructions:

- Preheat the oven to 400°F (200°C).
- Place salmon filet on a baking sheet and season with salt, pepper, and herbs.
- Toss sweet potato cubes and asparagus with olive oil, salt, and pepper.
- Arrange sweet potatoes and asparagus around the salmon.
- Cook in the oven for 20-25 minutes, or until the salmon is cooked through and the sweet potatoes are easily pierced with a fork.

Dessert: Dark Chocolate and Walnut Bites

Ingredients:

- 1 ounce dark chocolate (70% cocoa or higher for antioxidants)
- 1/4 cup walnuts (omega-3 fatty acids and protein)

Instructions:

- Melt dark chocolate and drizzle over walnuts.
- Let cool and harden before eating.

Implementing Personalized Nutrition in Daily Life

1. Meal Prep and Planning: Dedicate time each week to plan and prepare meals. This ensures you have healthy, genetic-optimized options available and reduces the likelihood of reaching for unhealthy convenience foods.

2. Variety and Balance: Keep your meals varied to ensure a broad spectrum of nutrients and prevent dietary monotony. Rotate different protein sources, vegetables, and healthy fats to keep meals interesting and nutritionally balanced.

3. Monitoring and Adjustment: Regularly monitor your health and well-being to see how your personalized diet is affecting you. Be open to adjusting your meal plans based on feedback from your body and any new genetic insights you may receive.

4. Professional Guidance: Work with a nutritionist or healthcare provider who understands genetic testing and personalized nutrition. They can provide tailored advice, help interpret genetic data, and ensure your diet supports your overall health goals.

Chapter 3: Cognitive Enhancement and Mental Performance

In the ever-evolving landscape of biohacking and personalized health, cognitive enhancement stands out as a particularly intriguing and promising field. The quest for improved mental performance has led to the development of various strategies, supplements, and technologies designed to optimize brain function, enhance memory, increase focus, and boost overall cognitive abilities. This chapter delves into the science and practice of cognitive enhancement, exploring both traditional and cutting-edge approaches to unlocking the full potential of the human mind.

The Science of Cognitive Enhancement

Cognitive enhancement refers to the augmentation of mental functions such as memory, attention, executive function, and creativity. It can be achieved through a combination of lifestyle changes, dietary modifications, supplements, and technological interventions. The foundation of cognitive enhancement lies in understanding the brain's complex neurochemistry and how various factors can influence cognitive processes.

1. Neuroplasticity: The brain's remarkable capacity to adapt and change by creating new connections between brain cells, allowing it to reorganize and refine its function throughout a person's lifetime. Engaging in activities that challenge the brain, such as learning new skills, solving puzzles, or engaging in creative pursuits, can promote neuroplasticity, enhancing cognitive function.

2. Neurotransmitters: Chemical messengers in the brain, known as neurotransmitters, play a crucial role in regulating mood, focus, and cognitive abilities. For example, dopamine is associated with motivation and reward, while acetylcholine is involved in learning and memory. Balancing neurotransmitter levels through diet, supplements, and lifestyle choices can significantly impact cognitive performance.

3. Brain-Derived Neurotrophic Factor (BDNF): BDNF is a protein that supports the survival, growth, and differentiation of neurons. Higher levels of BDNF are linked to improved cognitive function and mental health. Exercise, a healthy diet, and certain supplements can increase BDNF levels, promoting brain health and cognitive enhancement.

Traditional Approaches to Cognitive Enhancement

1. Nutrition and Diet: A well-balanced diet rich in essential nutrients is fundamental to cognitive health. Antioxidant-rich foods, such as berries and leafy greens, protect the brain from oxidative stress. Additionally, vitamins and minerals like B vitamins, vitamin D, and magnesium support cognitive processes.

2. Exercise: Physical activity has a profound impact on brain health. Regular exercise increases blood flow to the brain, promotes neuroplasticity, and boosts the production of BDNF. Aerobic exercises, such as running and swimming, are particularly beneficial for cognitive function.

3. Sleep: Quality sleep is essential for memory consolidation, emotional regulation, and overall cognitive performance. Establishing a regular sleep schedule, creating a restful sleep environment, and practicing good sleep hygiene can enhance mental performance.

4. Mindfulness and Meditation: Mindfulness practices and meditation have been shown to improve attention, reduce stress, and enhance cognitive flexibility. These practices can increase gray matter in brain regions associated with learning and memory, leading to better cognitive function.

Cutting-Edge Approaches to Cognitive Enhancement

1. Nootropics: Nootropics, also known as smart drugs or cognitive enhancers, are substances that can improve cognitive function. These include natural supplements like ginkgo biloba, bacopa monnieri, and Rhodiola rosea, as well as synthetic compounds like racetams and modafinil. Nootropics can enhance memory, focus, and mental clarity, though their effectiveness varies among individuals.

2. Neurofeedback: Neurofeedback is a form of biofeedback that uses real-time monitoring of brain activity to teach self-regulation of brain function. By providing feedback on brainwave patterns, individuals can learn to modulate their brain activity, leading to improved cognitive performance and emotional regulation.

3. Transcranial Direct Current Stimulation (tDCS): tDCS is a non-invasive brain stimulation technique that uses low electrical currents to modulate neuronal activity. It has shown promise in enhancing cognitive functions such as working memory, attention, and problem-solving skills. While tDCS is still under research, it offers potential as a tool for cognitive enhancement.

4. Genetic Interventions: Advances in genetic research have opened the door to potential cognitive enhancement through genetic interventions. Identifying and modifying genes associated with cognitive function could lead to personalized approaches for optimizing mental performance. While this field is still in its infancy, it holds significant promise for the future.

Case Studies and Real-World Applications

To illustrate the practical application of cognitive enhancement strategies, consider the case of Sarah, a 40-year-old professional facing cognitive decline and reduced mental clarity. After undergoing genetic testing, Sarah discovered that she had a genetic predisposition to lower BDNF levels and slower dopamine metabolism. With this information, Sarah embarked on a personalized cognitive enhancement plan that included:

1. **Dietary Adjustments:** Sarah increased her intake of omega-3 fatty acids by incorporating more fatty fish and flaxseeds into her diet. She also included antioxidant-rich foods and supplements to support brain health.

2. **Exercise Routine:** Sarah began a regular aerobic exercise regimen, including jogging and swimming, to boost BDNF levels and improve overall brain function.

3. **Mindfulness Practices:** She integrated mindfulness meditation into her daily routine to enhance focus, reduce stress, and improve cognitive flexibility.

4. **Nootropic Supplements:** Based on her genetic profile, Sarah started taking specific nootropic supplements, including bacopa monnieri and Rhodiola rosea, to enhance memory and mental clarity.

After several months, Sarah experienced significant improvements in her cognitive function, including better memory, increased focus, and enhanced mental clarity.

Her personalized approach to cognitive enhancement demonstrated the potential of combining traditional and cutting-edge strategies for optimal brain health.

Nootropics: The Brain Boosters

Nootropics, often referred to as "smart drugs" or "cognitive enhancers," have garnered significant attention in the realm of biohacking and personalized health. These substances aim to improve mental skills like memory, creativity, and focus, helping people think and perform better. As the desire for enhanced mental performance grows, nootropics offer promising solutions for those looking to unlock their brain's full potential. This chapter explores the science behind nootropics, their benefits, types, and considerations for safe usage.

The Science Behind Nootropics

The word 'nootropic' was first introduced in the 1970s by Dr. Corneliu E. Giurgea, a Romanian expert in psychology and chemistry, who derived it from the Greek words for 'mind' and 'to shape or influence', essentially meaning a substance that shapes or enhances the mind. According to Giurgea, a true nootropic must enhance learning and memory, protect the brain from physical or chemical injury, improve the efficacy of neuronal firing mechanisms, and possess few side effects.

Nootropics work through various mechanisms to boost brain function:

1. **Neurotransmitter Modulation:** Nootropics can influence the levels of neurotransmitters, such as acetylcholine, dopamine, serotonin, and glutamate, which play crucial roles in mood, attention, and memory.

2. **Neuroprotection:** Some nootropics have antioxidant and anti-inflammatory properties that protect the brain from oxidative stress and damage.

3. **Cerebral Blood Flow:** By enhancing blood flow to the brain, nootropics can improve oxygen and nutrient delivery, supporting cognitive processes.

4. **Neurogenesis and Neuroplasticity:** Certain nootropics stimulate the growth of new neurons and the formation of new neural connections, essential for learning and memory.

Benefits of Nootropics

1. Enhanced Memory and Learning: Nootropics like piracetam and bacopa monnieri have been shown to improve memory retention and recall, making them valuable for students and professionals alike.

2. Increased Focus and Attention: Stimulant nootropics, such as caffeine and modafinil, can enhance alertness and concentration, helping users stay productive for longer periods.

3. Improved Mood and Reduced Anxiety: Nootropics like L-theanine and Rhodiola rosea promote relaxation and reduce stress, leading to a more balanced emotional state.

4. Boosted Creativity: Certain nootropics, such as aniracetam, are believed to enhance creative thinking and problem-solving abilities.

Types of Nootropics

Nootropics come in two main types: natural (found in nature) and synthetic (created in a lab).

1. Natural Nootropics:

• *Bacopa Monnieri:* An herbal supplement traditionally used in Ayurvedic medicine, known for enhancing memory and reducing anxiety.

• *Ginkgo Biloba:* An extract from the ginkgo tree, reputed to improve cognitive function and blood circulation in the brain.

• *Rhodiola Rosea:* An adaptogenic herb that helps combat fatigue and stress, improving mental clarity.

• *Lion's Mane Mushroom:* Known for its neuroprotective properties and ability to stimulate nerve growth factor (NGF), promoting neurogenesis.

2. Synthetic Nootropics:

• *Piracetam:* One of the first and most studied nootropics, piracetam enhances cognitive function and memory.

• *Modafinil:* A prescription drug that promotes wakefulness and is used to treat narcolepsy. It's also popular among those seeking to enhance focus and productivity.

• *Aniracetam:* Known for its cognitive-enhancing and anxiolytic properties, aniracetam improves memory and reduces anxiety.

- ***Noopept:*** A powerful synthetic nootropic that enhances memory, learning, and overall cognitive function, often considered more potent than piracetam.

Safety and Considerations

While nootropics offer potential cognitive benefits, their safety and efficacy can vary widely. It's crucial to exercise careful consideration and restraint when using nootropics.

1. **Research and Quality:** Ensure that you are using well-researched and high-quality nootropics. Look for products from reputable manufacturers and check for third-party testing.

2. **Dosage:** Follow recommended dosages and start with the lowest effective dose to assess your tolerance. Using nootropics excessively or improperly can result in harmful consequences.

3. **Consultation:** Before starting any nootropic regimen, consult with a healthcare professional, especially if you have underlying health conditions or are taking other medications.

4. Monitoring: Keep track of your response to nootropics, noting any positive or negative effects. Adjust your regimen accordingly and discontinue use if adverse effects occur.

Chapter 4: Fitness Tailored to Your Genes

Tailoring fitness programs to an individual's genetic profile represents a cutting-edge approach to achieving optimal physical performance and well-being. The intersection of genetics and fitness offers a transformative way to understand how our bodies respond to different types of exercise, recovery, and nutrition. By decoding our genetic blueprint, we can design customized fitness plans that maximize results and minimize injury risk. This chapter delves into the science of genetic fitness profiling, its benefits, and how to apply these insights for a truly personalized fitness regimen.

The Science of Genetic Fitness Profiling

Genetic fitness profiling involves analyzing specific genes related to physical performance, recovery, and injury susceptibility. Advances in genetic testing have made it possible to identify variations in these genes, providing valuable insights into how our bodies are likely to respond to different types of exercise. Some key areas of focus include:

1. Muscle Fiber Composition: Genes like ACTN3 and ACE influence whether you are predisposed to having more fast-twitch or slow-twitch muscle fibers. Fast-twitch fibers are associated with explosive power and strength, ideal for activities like sprinting and weightlifting. Slow-twitch fibers, on the other hand, are more efficient for endurance activities like long-distance running.

2. Aerobic Capacity and VO2 Max: The PPARGC1A gene plays a role in mitochondrial biogenesis, affecting aerobic capacity and endurance performance. Understanding your genetic predisposition can help tailor cardio training to improve oxygen utilization and stamina.

3. Recovery and Injury Risk: Genes such as COL1A1 and COL5A1 influence collagen production, affecting ligament and tendon strength. Variations in these genes can indicate a higher risk of injuries like tendonitis or ligament tears. Additionally, genes related to inflammation and oxidative stress can inform recovery strategies, ensuring optimal rest and repair.

4. Metabolism and Nutrient Utilization: Genetic variations in the FTO and MTHFR genes, among others, can impact how efficiently your body metabolizes fats, carbohydrates, and proteins. This information can guide nutritional choices to support your fitness goals, whether it's building muscle, losing fat, or improving endurance.

Benefits of Tailored Fitness Programs

1. Optimized Training: By understanding your genetic predispositions, you can design a training program that leverages your strengths and addresses your weaknesses. For example, if you have a higher proportion of fast-twitch fibers, incorporating more high-intensity interval training (HIIT) and strength training can maximize your performance.

2. Injury Prevention: Knowing your genetic susceptibility to injuries allows you to take proactive measures to prevent them. This might include specific warm-up routines, targeted strength exercises, or recovery strategies tailored to your genetic profile.

3. Enhanced Recovery: Personalized insights into how your body recovers from exercise can inform better recovery protocols. Whether it's adjusting your rest periods, incorporating specific anti-inflammatory foods, or using recovery techniques like cryotherapy or massage, you can optimize recovery and reduce downtime.

4. Effective Nutrition: Tailoring your diet to your genetic profile ensures you are fueling your body in the most efficient way possible. Understanding your unique nutrient needs can help you avoid deficiencies, improve performance, and accelerate recovery.

Applying Genetic Insights to Your Fitness Regimen

1. Genetic Testing: The first step in tailoring your fitness program to your genes is undergoing genetic testing. Several companies offer DNA testing kits that analyze genes related to fitness and health. Once you receive your results, consult with a genetic counselor or a fitness expert with experience in genetic profiling to interpret the data.

2. Customized Training Plan: Based on your genetic profile, design a training plan that aligns with your strengths and addresses your weaknesses. For example, if you have a genetic predisposition for endurance, incorporate more long-distance running or cycling into your routine. Conversely, if you excel in power and strength, focus on resistance training and short, high-intensity workouts.

3. Injury Prevention Strategies: Use your genetic insights to identify areas of vulnerability and implement preventive measures. This could include specific exercises to strengthen weak areas, using proper techniques, and ensuring adequate rest and recovery.

4. Optimized Recovery Protocols: Tailor your recovery strategies to your genetic profile. If you have a higher propensity for inflammation, incorporate anti-inflammatory foods and supplements into your diet. Use recovery techniques like foam rolling, stretching, and active recovery sessions to promote healing and reduce the risk of injury.

5. Personalized Nutrition: Align your diet with your genetic predispositions to optimize performance and recovery. If your genes indicate a higher need for certain nutrients, adjust your diet to include foods rich in those nutrients or consider supplementation. Balance macronutrients according to your metabolic profile to ensure you are fueling your workouts effectively.

Case Study: Genetic Fitness Success

To illustrate the power of genetically tailored fitness programs, consider the case of John, a 35-year-old avid runner who struggled with recurrent injuries and plateaued performance. After undergoing genetic testing, John discovered he had a higher proportion of slow-twitch muscle fibers, making him naturally suited for endurance sports. However, he also had genetic markers indicating a higher risk for tendon injuries and slower recovery.

With these insights, John worked with a fitness expert to redesign his training program. He incorporated more long-distance running and reduced the intensity of his sprints, which had been causing undue strain on his tendons. He also added specific strength training exercises to support his tendons and ligaments. For recovery, John included more anti-inflammatory foods in his diet and practiced active recovery techniques.

Within a few months, John noticed significant improvements. His performance in long-distance events improved, and he experienced fewer injuries. By aligning his fitness regimen with his genetic profile, John unlocked his full potential and achieved his personal best times in marathons.

Designing a Workout Plan Based on Your Genetics

Designing a workout plan based on your genetics represents the pinnacle of personalized fitness. By leveraging insights from genetic testing, you can create a regimen that aligns with your unique physiological makeup, optimizing performance, reducing injury risk, and ensuring sustainable progress. This approach moves beyond the one-size-fits-all methodology, embracing a customized strategy that caters to your individual needs and capabilities. Here's how you can design a workout plan tailored to your genetics.

Understanding Your Genetic Profile

The first step in designing a genetically tailored workout plan is to undergo genetic testing. Various companies offer at-home DNA testing kits that analyze genes related to physical performance, muscle composition, endurance, recovery, and injury susceptibility. Once you have your results, you can interpret the data with the help of a genetic counselor or a fitness professional with experience in genetic profiling. Key genetic markers to consider include:

1. Muscle Fiber Type (ACTN3 and ACE Genes): These genes indicate whether you have a higher proportion of fast-twitch or slow-twitch muscle fibers. Fast-twitch fibers are ideal for explosive movements and strength activities, while slow-twitch fibers are better suited for endurance exercises.

2. Aerobic Capacity (PPARGC1A Gene): This gene affects your body's ability to produce energy aerobically, which is crucial for endurance activities. A high aerobic capacity means your body is efficient at using oxygen during prolonged exercise.

3. Recovery and Injury Risk (COL1A1 and COL5A1 Genes): These genes influence the strength and elasticity of your tendons and ligaments. Understanding your predisposition to injuries can help you implement preventive measures and optimize recovery strategies.

4. Metabolism and Nutrient Utilization (FTO and MTHFR Genes): These genes impact how your body metabolizes different macronutrients and processes certain vitamins. Tailoring your diet to complement your genetic makeup can enhance your workout performance and recovery.

Creating Your Customized Workout Plan

1. Strength Training: If your genetic profile indicates a higher proportion of fast-twitch muscle fibers (ACTN3), focus on strength and power-based exercises. Incorporate heavy lifting with lower repetitions and longer rest periods. Exercises like squats, deadlifts, bench presses, and Olympic lifts will leverage your natural predisposition for power. For those with more slow-twitch fibers, incorporate higher repetitions with moderate weights, focusing on endurance and muscular endurance.

2. Cardiovascular Training: For individuals with a high aerobic capacity (PPARGC1A), incorporate long-distance running, cycling, or swimming into your routine. These activities will maximize your endurance capabilities. If your aerobic capacity is lower, focus on high-intensity interval training (HIIT) to improve cardiovascular fitness and burn fat efficiently. HIIT workouts combine short bursts of intense activity with periods of rest or low-intensity exercise, catering to both fast and slow-twitch fibers.

3. Flexibility and Mobility: Incorporate stretching and mobility exercises to enhance flexibility and prevent injuries. If your genetic profile shows a higher risk of ligament or tendon injuries (COL1A1 and COL5A1), prioritize exercises that strengthen these areas, such as dynamic stretches, yoga, or Pilates. Regular flexibility training can improve your range of motion and reduce the likelihood of injuries.

4. Recovery Protocols: Tailor your recovery strategies based on your genetic predisposition to inflammation and oxidative stress. If you have genes indicating slower recovery, integrate practices like foam rolling, massage, and cryotherapy into your routine. Emphasize proper hydration, sleep, and nutrition to support recovery. Consuming anti-inflammatory foods, such as berries, fatty fish, and leafy greens, can help mitigate inflammation and promote healing.

5. Nutrition and Supplementation: Align your diet with your genetic profile to fuel your workouts effectively. If your genes suggest a higher need for certain nutrients (FTO and MTHFR), adjust your diet accordingly. Ensure a balanced intake of macronutrients—proteins, fats, and carbohydrates—to support your training goals. Consider supplementation if necessary, but consult with a healthcare professional before starting any new supplements.

Tracking and Adjusting Your Plan

Once your genetically tailored workout plan is in place, monitor your progress regularly. Keep track of your performance, recovery, and any signs of injury or fatigue. Use wearable fitness trackers, apps, or a fitness journal to log your workouts and recovery metrics. Based on your observations and feedback, adjust your plan to optimize results. This iterative approach ensures that your workout regimen evolves with your changing needs and goals.

Recovery and Injury Prevention Personalized

In today's world of advanced fitness and health, one-size-fits-all approaches to recovery and injury prevention are rapidly becoming outdated. Personalized strategies, tailored to individual genetic profiles, offer a more effective way to enhance performance, reduce downtime, and prevent injuries. By understanding your body's unique needs, you can optimize your recovery process and safeguard yourself against potential injuries, ensuring longevity in your fitness journey. Here's how personalized recovery and injury prevention can revolutionize your approach to health and fitness.

The Impact of Genetics on Recovery and Injury

Your genetic makeup plays a significant role in how your body responds to exercise, heals from stress, and recovers from injuries. Specific genes influence how quickly you recover, your susceptibility to certain injuries, and your body's inflammatory response. For instance:

1. Inflammation and Healing (IL6 and TNF Genes): These genes regulate the body's inflammatory response. Variations in these genes can determine how much inflammation you experience after intense exercise, which directly impacts recovery time and injury risk.

2. Tendon and Ligament Strength (COL1A1 and COL5A1 Genes): These genes are associated with the production of collagen, a key component of tendons and ligaments. Genetic variations can influence the strength and elasticity of these tissues, affecting your susceptibility to injuries like tendonitis or ligament tears.

3. Muscle Recovery (ACTN3 Gene): The ACTN3 gene, often referred to as the "sprinter gene," influences muscle composition and recovery. Depending on the variant you carry, you may have a natural advantage in either endurance or power sports, and this can also affect how your muscles recover after exercise.

Personalized Recovery Strategies

Understanding your genetic predispositions allows you to create a recovery plan tailored to your specific needs:

1. Anti-Inflammatory Nutrition: If your genetic profile suggests a heightened inflammatory response, incorporating anti-inflammatory foods into your diet can be highly beneficial. Omega-3 fatty acids, found in fish like salmon, and antioxidants from berries, leafy greens, and nuts, can help mitigate inflammation and speed up recovery.

2. Optimized Sleep: Sleep is crucial for recovery, and genetics can influence your sleep patterns. The CLOCK gene, for example, regulates circadian rhythms. If your genetic profile indicates sleep challenges, you might benefit from creating a consistent sleep routine, using blue light filters in the evening, and practicing relaxation techniques like meditation before bed.

3. Active Recovery Techniques: Personalized active recovery strategies can be incredibly effective. For those with a genetic tendency toward slower muscle recovery, incorporating low-intensity activities like swimming, walking, or yoga can help maintain blood flow and promote healing without adding additional strain on the body.

Tailored Injury Prevention

Injury prevention becomes significantly more effective when it's tailored to your genetic risks:

1. Targeted Strengthening: If you are genetically predisposed to weaker tendons or ligaments, incorporating targeted strengthening exercises is essential. Eccentric exercises, which involve lengthening a muscle under tension (such as the lowering phase of a bicep curl), can help strengthen these connective tissues and reduce injury risk.

2. Flexibility and Mobility: Genetics can also influence your natural flexibility and joint health. Regularly practicing flexibility and mobility exercises, such as dynamic stretching and foam rolling, can help prevent injuries by maintaining joint range of motion and muscle elasticity.

3. Proper Warm-Up and Cool-Down: Personalized warm-up and cool-down routines are critical. For example, if your genetic profile indicates a higher risk of muscle stiffness, you should spend extra time warming up with dynamic movements that mimic your workout. Cooling down with static stretches can also help reduce post-workout stiffness and promote faster recovery.

Monitoring and Adjusting Your Plan

Your body's response to exercise and recovery isn't static, and neither should your approach be. Regularly monitoring how your body feels and performs can help you fine-tune your recovery and injury prevention strategies. Tools like fitness trackers, apps, and even simple journaling can provide valuable insights into what works best for you.

Chapter 5: Mental Health and Emotional Resilience

As we navigate daily stressors and life's inevitable challenges, building and maintaining mental well-being is essential not just for personal fulfillment but also for our overall health. Chapter 8 delves into the vital role that mental health and emotional resilience play in biohacking and personalized health, exploring strategies that can empower individuals to thrive in an often overwhelming world.

Understanding Mental Health and Emotional Resilience

Mental health encompasses our emotional, psychological, and social well-being. It influences how we think, feel, and act, affecting every aspect of our lives, from how we handle stress to how we relate to others and make decisions. Emotional resilience, on the other hand, refers to the ability to adapt to stressful situations and bounce back from adversity. While resilience doesn't eliminate stress or erase life's difficulties, it provides the strength to deal with them in a way that fosters recovery and growth.

For years, mental health has been a somewhat overlooked aspect of overall well-being, often overshadowed by physical health. However, the growing recognition of its significance, coupled with advances in personalized health, has brought mental wellness to the forefront. Understanding the intricate connection between the mind and body is key to achieving true health and resilience.

The Science of Mental Health: Genetics and Environment

Mental health is influenced by a complex interplay of genetics, environment, and lifestyle choices. Certain genetic factors can predispose individuals to mental health conditions such as anxiety, depression, and bipolar disorder. However, genetics is only part of the equation; environmental factors such as childhood experiences, trauma, and even socioeconomic status play a significant role in shaping mental health outcomes.

Recent advancements in genetic testing allow for a deeper understanding of one's predisposition to mental health challenges. For instance, variations in genes related to neurotransmitter production and regulation (such as the serotonin transporter gene, 5-HTTLPR) can affect mood regulation and stress response. Armed with this knowledge, individuals can adopt targeted strategies to manage stress, enhance mental resilience, and improve overall well-being.

Building Emotional Resilience: Personalized Strategies

Emotional resilience can be cultivated, and like physical fitness, it requires regular practice and commitment. Here are personalized strategies to enhance emotional resilience:

1. Mindfulness and Meditation: These practices help cultivate present-moment awareness, reduce stress, and increase emotional regulation. Mindfulness techniques, such as deep breathing and meditation, can rewire the brain to become more resilient to stress. Personalized meditation practices, based on individual needs and preferences, can further enhance these benefits, making it easier to integrate into daily life.

2. Cognitive Behavioral Therapy (CBT): CBT is a widely recognized approach to managing mental health challenges by addressing negative thought patterns and behaviors. Personalized CBT can be more effective when it takes into account an individual's specific triggers and thought processes. Working with a therapist who tailors the approach to your unique needs can lead to significant improvements in emotional resilience.

3. Social Support Networks: Strong social connections are crucial for mental health and emotional resilience. Personalized strategies for building and maintaining these networks include identifying and nurturing relationships that provide emotional support, as well as setting healthy boundaries to protect one's mental well-being.

4. Physical Activity: Regular exercise is not only beneficial for physical health but also for mental well-being. Physical activity releases endorphins, the body's natural mood lifters, and can reduce symptoms of depression and anxiety. Personalized fitness plans that cater to individual preferences and genetic predispositions can maximize the mental health benefits of exercise.

5. Healthy Sleep Habits: Sleep is fundamental to mental health. Poor sleep can exacerbate mental health issues, while good sleep hygiene supports emotional resilience. Personalized sleep strategies might include optimizing your environment for sleep, creating a bedtime routine, and using technology mindfully to avoid overstimulation before bed.

6. Nutrition for the Mind: Diet plays a significant role in mental health. Nutritional psychiatry is an emerging field that explores how food affects mood and cognitive function. Personalized nutrition plans that take into account genetic predispositions to certain nutrient deficiencies or intolerances can help support mental health. For example, diets rich in omega-3 fatty acids, vitamins B6 and B12, and magnesium have been linked to improved mood and reduced anxiety.

Case Study: Tailoring Mental Health Strategies

Consider the example of James, a 35-year-old software engineer who struggled with chronic anxiety. After undergoing genetic testing, James discovered he had a variation in the COMT gene, which affects dopamine metabolism and is associated with stress sensitivity. With this insight, James worked with a mental health professional to develop a personalized strategy that included mindfulness meditation tailored to his high-stress environment, a customized exercise regimen focusing on stress relief, and a diet plan rich in nutrients known to support dopamine regulation.

Over time, James noticed significant improvements in his anxiety levels and overall mental well-being. His personalized approach to mental health allowed him to build emotional resilience, leading to greater satisfaction in both his personal and professional life.

Enhancing Mood and Emotional Well-being

Emotional well-being is the cornerstone of overall health, influencing not only our mental state but also our physical health, relationships, and productivity.

Enhancing mood and emotional well-being involves a holistic approach that integrates lifestyle choices, mental health practices, and an understanding of individual needs. This chapter explores strategies for improving mood and emotional resilience, offering insights into how personalized approaches can lead to a more balanced and fulfilling life.

Understanding Mood and Emotional Well-being

Mood is a temporary state of mind that can be influenced by various factors, including stress, environment, diet, physical activity, and even genetics. Emotional well-being, on the other hand, refers to the broader state of being content, having a positive self-image, and feeling balanced emotionally. While fluctuations in mood are normal, consistently low mood or emotional instability can lead to more serious mental health issues such as anxiety or depression.

The key to enhancing mood and emotional well-being lies in recognizing the interconnectedness of the mind and body. Physical health, mental health, and emotional well-being are deeply intertwined, and improving one often leads to improvements in the others. For instance, regular physical activity can boost mood through the release of endorphins, while a balanced diet can influence brain chemistry and emotional stability.

The Science Behind Mood Regulation

Mood regulation is a complex process governed by various neurotransmitters in the brain, including serotonin, dopamine, and norepinephrine. These chemicals play a crucial role in how we feel, think, and respond to stress. For example, serotonin is often referred to as the "feel-good" neurotransmitter because it helps regulate mood, appetite, and sleep. Dopamine is associated with pleasure and reward, influencing motivation and feelings of happiness. Norepinephrine helps the body respond to stress and plays a role in mood regulation.

Genetic variations can affect how these neurotransmitters function, which can influence mood and emotional well-being. For instance, certain variations in the serotonin transporter gene (5-HTTLPR) have been linked to an increased risk of depression.

Understanding these genetic factors can provide valuable insights into personalized strategies for mood enhancement.

Personalized Strategies for Enhancing Mood

1. Nutrition for a Healthy Mind: Diet plays a significant role in mood regulation. For example, tryptophan, an amino acid found in foods like turkey, eggs, and nuts, is a precursor to serotonin. Omega-3 fatty acids, found in fish like salmon and sardines, are known to support brain health and reduce symptoms of depression. A personalized nutrition plan that addresses specific nutrient deficiencies or genetic predispositions can significantly impact mood and emotional well-being.

2. Exercise and Physical Activity: Regular physical activity is one of the most effective ways to enhance mood. Additionally, physical activity increases dopamine production, leading to improved motivation and feelings of pleasure. A personalized fitness plan that aligns with an individual's preferences and genetic makeup can maximize these benefits, making it easier to maintain a consistent exercise routine.

3. Mindfulness and Meditation: Mindfulness practices such as meditation, deep breathing, and progressive muscle relaxation can help regulate emotions and reduce stress. These techniques train the mind to focus on the present moment, reducing the impact of negative thoughts and emotions. Personalized mindfulness practices, tailored to individual stressors and emotional needs, can be particularly effective in enhancing mood and emotional well-being.

4. Sleep Hygiene: Sleep is essential for mood regulation. Poor sleep can exacerbate feelings of anxiety, depression, and irritability, while quality sleep can enhance emotional resilience and mood stability. Personalized sleep strategies might include creating a consistent bedtime routine, optimizing the sleep environment, and addressing any genetic predispositions to sleep disturbances.

5. Social Connections: Human beings are inherently social creatures, and strong social connections are vital for emotional well-being. Engaging in meaningful relationships and building a support network can provide emotional stability and improve mood. For those who may struggle with social anxiety or introversion, personalized strategies for building and maintaining relationships can help create a supportive and enriching social environment.

6. Cognitive Behavioral Techniques: Cognitive Behavioral Therapy (CBT) is an evidence-based approach to managing mood disorders by addressing negative thought patterns. Personalized CBT can help individuals identify and challenge cognitive distortions that contribute to low mood, replacing them with healthier, more balanced thoughts. This process not only improves mood but also enhances emotional resilience.

Case Study: Personalized Mood Enhancement

Consider the example of Emily, a 40-year-old marketing professional who struggled with persistent low mood and stress. After undergoing genetic testing, Emily discovered she had a variation in the 5-HTTLPR gene, which affected her serotonin levels. With this knowledge, Emily and her therapist developed a personalized mood enhancement plan. This plan included a diet rich in tryptophan and omega-3 fatty acids, a regular exercise routine focusing on activities she enjoyed, and mindfulness practices tailored to her work-related stressors.

Over several months, Emily noticed significant improvements in her mood and emotional well-being. Her personalized approach allowed her to address the underlying factors contributing to her low mood, leading to greater emotional stability and a more positive outlook on life.

Conclusion: Embracing the Biohacking Lifestyle

The concept of biohacking may seem futuristic or even intimidating, but at its core, it is about taking control of your own health and well-being in a deeply personalized way. By leveraging advances in science and technology, biohacking allows you to make informed decisions about your body, mind, and environment to enhance your quality of life. As we've explored throughout this book, biohacking encompasses a wide range of practices—from optimizing your diet and fitness based on your genetic profile to enhancing cognitive performance and emotional resilience through targeted strategies.

Embracing the biohacking lifestyle is not about quick fixes or following fads; it is a journey of continuous self-improvement and self-discovery. It involves a commitment to understanding how your unique biology interacts with the world around you, and how you can make changes to live a healthier, longer, and more fulfilling life. Here's how you can start embracing the biohacking lifestyle in a sustainable and meaningful way.

1. Start with Awareness

The first step in any biohacking journey is awareness. This means developing a deep understanding of your body, mind, and environment. Biohacking begins with asking questions: How does your body respond to different foods? What exercises make you feel your best? How does your sleep pattern affect your mood and productivity? By becoming more aware of these interactions, you can start to identify areas where you want to make changes.

This awareness often involves collecting data about yourself. This could be as simple as keeping a health journal or using wearable technology to track your sleep, activity levels, and heart rate. For those interested in more in-depth exploration, genetic testing can offer insights into your unique biological makeup, revealing predispositions that can guide your biohacking strategies.

2. Experiment with Small Changes

Biohacking doesn't require a complete overhaul of your lifestyle overnight. In fact, one of the most effective ways to embrace biohacking is through small, incremental changes. Start by experimenting with one area of your life, such as nutrition, fitness, or sleep. For example, you might try adjusting your diet to include more foods that support brain health, or you might experiment with different exercise routines to see which one boosts your energy levels the most.

The key to successful biohacking is to approach these changes with curiosity and an open mind. Not every experiment will yield positive results, and that's okay. The process of trial and error is a fundamental part of biohacking. By making small, manageable changes and observing how your body responds, you can gradually build a lifestyle that is truly tailored to your individual needs.

3. Personalize Your Approach

One of the central tenets of biohacking is personalization. What works for one person may not work for another, and the beauty of biohacking is that it empowers you to discover what works best for you. Personalization can take many forms, from adjusting your diet based on genetic insights to developing a fitness routine that aligns with your body's strengths and weaknesses.

The personalization aspect of biohacking also extends to mental and emotional well-being. For example, while meditation might be the perfect stress-relief tool for some, others might find that physical activity or creative expression better supports their mental health. The goal is to create a personalized toolkit of practices that enhance your overall well-being.

4. Prioritize Sustainability

Biohacking is most effective when it is sustainable over the long term. This means choosing practices and habits that you can realistically maintain as part of your daily life. While some biohacks might involve temporary or intense interventions (such as fasting or high-intensity training), it's important to balance these with sustainable habits that support your health in the long run.

Sustainability also involves recognizing the importance of rest and recovery. The biohacking lifestyle is not about pushing yourself to the limit at all times; it's about finding a rhythm that allows for growth and renewal. By prioritizing practices that nourish your body and mind, you can maintain the benefits of biohacking over the years.

5. Embrace the Journey

Finally, embracing the biohacking lifestyle means seeing it as a journey rather than a destination. There is always more to learn, more to explore, and more ways to optimize your health and well-being. The field of biohacking is constantly evolving, with new research and technologies emerging all the time. By staying curious and open to new ideas, you can continue to refine and enhance your biohacking practices.

This journey is deeply personal, and it's important to celebrate the progress you make along the way.

Whether it's improved energy levels, better mental clarity, or enhanced physical performance, each small victory is a step toward a healthier, more fulfilling life.

Reflecting on Your Journey

As you reach the conclusion of your biohacking journey, it's important to take a moment to reflect on how far you've come. Biohacking is not just about the physical changes you've made or the new habits you've cultivated—it's about the deeper understanding of yourself that you've gained along the way. Reflecting on your journey allows you to appreciate the progress you've made, recognize the challenges you've overcome, and set the stage for continued growth and exploration.

Recognizing Your Achievements

One of the most rewarding aspects of biohacking is seeing tangible results from the changes you've implemented. Whether it's improved energy levels, better sleep, enhanced cognitive function, or a stronger sense of emotional well-being, it's crucial to acknowledge these achievements. Reflecting on your journey means celebrating these victories, no matter how small they may seem. Each improvement is a testament to your commitment to your health and well-being, and taking the time to recognize these milestones reinforces your motivation to continue.

Consider the specific goals you set when you first began biohacking. Perhaps you wanted to optimize your diet, increase your physical fitness, or manage stress more effectively. Reflecting on these initial goals and how they have evolved over time can give you a sense of accomplishment. You may find that you've surpassed your original expectations, or you might discover new goals that have emerged as a result of your progress. Either way, recognizing your achievements is an essential part of your biohacking journey.

Learning from Challenges

No journey is without its challenges, and biohacking is no exception. There may have been moments of frustration, setbacks, or even doubts about whether certain changes were making a difference. Reflecting on these challenges is just as important as celebrating your successes. These experiences provide valuable insights into your limits, preferences, and areas where you may need to adjust your approach.

For example, you might have tried a particular diet or exercise routine that didn't yield the results you expected. Rather than seeing this as a failure, reflect on what you learned from the experience. Perhaps it taught you more about your body's unique needs or helped you discover a different approach that worked better for you. Challenges are an inevitable part of any growth process, and by reflecting on them, you can transform them into opportunities for learning and self-improvement.

Embracing Continuous Growth

Reflecting on your biohacking journey also involves recognizing that this journey is ongoing. Biohacking is not a one-time effort but a lifelong commitment to optimizing your health and well-being. As you reflect, think about the areas where you still see potential for growth. What new goals do you want to pursue? What aspects of your health or lifestyle are you curious to explore next?

Continuous growth means staying open to new information, techniques, and technologies that can further enhance your well-being. The field of biohacking is constantly evolving, and as new research emerges, there will always be new opportunities to refine and expand your approach. Reflecting on your journey allows you to assess where you are now and where you want to go next, ensuring that you continue to evolve along with your goals.

Looking Back, Moving Forward

Finally, reflecting on your biohacking journey is a time to appreciate the broader impact it has had on your life. How has biohacking changed the way you view your health, your body, and your potential? Have you developed a deeper connection to your own well-being? Reflecting on these questions can help you understand the significance of the journey you've undertaken and the profound ways it has shaped your life.

As you move forward, carry with you the lessons, achievements, and insights you've gained. Your biohacking journey is a powerful example of what's possible when you take control of your health and make intentional, informed decisions about your well-being. By reflecting on your progress, you set the foundation for a future filled with continued growth, discovery, and empowerment.

Appendix: Resources and Further Reading

The world of biohacking and personalized health is vast, continuously evolving, and rich with resources for those who wish to dive deeper into the subject. As you continue your journey toward optimizing your health and well-being, having access to reliable, well-researched, and diverse resources will empower you to make informed decisions. This appendix provides a curated list of resources—ranging from books and scientific journals to websites, podcasts, and online communities—that will help you expand your knowledge and stay updated on the latest developments in biohacking.

Books

Books remain one of the most comprehensive ways to explore complex topics like biohacking. The following are essential reads that offer both foundational knowledge and cutting-edge insights:

1. "The Body Keeps the Score" by Bessel van der Kolk

This seminal work explores the profound connection between mind and body, delving into how trauma and stress can manifest physically. It's an invaluable resource for understanding the importance of emotional well-being in the context of biohacking.

2. "Deep Work" by Cal Newport

Newport's book is essential for anyone looking to enhance cognitive performance and mental clarity. It offers strategies for focusing in a distracted world, making it a key resource for the cognitive enhancement side of biohacking.

Scientific Journals and Articles

For those who want to delve into the latest research, scientific journals and articles are indispensable. Access to peer-reviewed studies ensures that you are basing your biohacking practices on the most reliable information available.

1. Nature Biotechnology

This journal offers cutting-edge research on the intersection of biology and technology. It's an excellent resource for staying informed about the latest advancements that may influence future biohacking techniques.

2. The Journal of Personalized Medicine

As personalized health becomes more mainstream, this journal provides comprehensive coverage of innovations in genomics, pharmacogenomics, and individualized care strategies. It's ideal for those interested in the scientific underpinnings of personalized health.

3. PubMed (www.pubmed.gov)

An online database of medical research, PubMed is a treasure trove of peer-reviewed articles on every imaginable aspect of health. Whether you're researching specific genes or looking for studies on the effectiveness of nootropics, PubMed is an invaluable resource.

Websites and Online Platforms

The internet is a dynamic space for biohacking enthusiasts, offering everything from forums and blogs to educational platforms and online courses.

1. Bulletproof (www.bulletproof.com)

Founded by Dave Asprey, one of the pioneers of the biohacking movement, Bulletproof's website offers a wealth of articles, podcasts, and product recommendations. It's particularly useful for those interested in the intersection of nutrition, performance, and longevity.

2. Quantified Self (www.quantifiedself.com)

This online community is dedicated to self-tracking and data-driven personal experimentation. The site offers a range of tools, articles, and event information for those who want to delve deeper into the quantification side of biohacking.

3. Mindvalley (www.mindvalley.com)

Mindvalley provides online courses and content that blend science with spiritual practices, focusing on personal growth, health, and well-being. It's a valuable resource for biohackers interested in the holistic integration of mind, body, and spirit.

Podcasts

Podcasts offer a flexible and accessible way to stay up-to-date and motivated, even when you're on the move.

Here are a few that regularly feature discussions on biohacking, personalized health, and cutting-edge science:

1. "The Tim Ferriss Show"

Tim Ferriss is known for his deep dives into self-improvement, productivity, and health. His podcast features interviews with experts across various fields, including biohacking pioneers, making it a must-listen for anyone interested in personal optimization.

2. "The Ben Greenfield Fitness Podcast"

Ben Greenfield is a well-known figure in the biohacking community. His podcast covers a broad range of topics, including fitness, nutrition, supplements, and cutting-edge biohacking techniques. It's an excellent resource for both beginners and seasoned biohackers.

3. "FoundMyFitness" with Dr. Rhonda Patrick

Dr. Rhonda Patrick's podcast is renowned for its in-depth discussions on nutrition, aging, and health optimization. Her interviews with leading scientists provide listeners with a robust understanding of the science behind biohacking practices.

Online Communities and Forums

Engaging with a community of like-minded individuals can provide support, inspiration, and new ideas for your biohacking journey. Here are a few online communities worth exploring:

1. Reddit – r/Biohackers

This subreddit is a thriving community where members share tips, experiences, and questions about all things biohacking. It's a great place to connect with others and learn from the collective knowledge of the community.

2. Health Optimization Summit (www.health optimization summit.com)

An annual event that gathers the world's leading health and biohacking experts, the Health Optimization Summit also has an active online presence where enthusiasts can connect, share, and learn throughout the year.

3. Facebook Groups

There are numerous Facebook groups dedicated to various aspects of biohacking, such as "Biohacking Secrets" and "Biohackers Lab." These groups offer a platform for sharing experiences, asking questions, and staying up to date with the latest trends and techniques.

Acknowledgments

This book would not have been possible without the support and inspiration of those who have been a part of my journey. To my family and friends, thank you for your unwavering belief in me. To the pioneers of biohacking, whose passion and innovation light the way—your work continues to inspire and challenge us all. And to you, the reader, for embracing the pursuit of a healthier, longer life. Here's to the future we're building together. Thank you.

About the Author

Garth E. Wells is a trailblazer in the world of biohacking and personalized health, known for his innovative approach to unlocking human potential. With a keen interest in the science of well-being, Garth has spent years pushing the boundaries of what's possible, transforming cutting-edge research into practical strategies for everyday life.

Driven by a passion for optimizing mind, body, and spirit, Garth's journey began with a simple question: How can we live healthier, longer, and more fulfilling lives? This curiosity led him to explore the depths of genetic science, nutrition, and mental performance, all while experimenting with the latest in health technology.

Today, Garth E. Wells is a sought-after expert and a trusted guide for those looking to elevate their lives through personalized health. His work inspires others to take charge of their well-being, offering a fresh perspective on what it means to truly thrive. When he's not writing or speaking, Garth continues to explore new frontiers in biohacking, always aiming to live—and help others live—at their full potential.